The solution to obesity:

Conquer Cravings, Shed Pounds, and Boost Vitality"

By

James L. Gardner

Table of content

Introduction

Consequences Of obesity

CHAPTER 1

WHAT CAUSED THE OBESITY EPIDERMIC?

CHAPTER 2

THE HORMONAL MECHANISM OF OBESITY

CHAPTER 3

THE CALORIE CONUNDRUM

CHAPTER 4

STRUCTURING A DIET FOR SUSTAINABLE WEIGHT LOSS

Introduction

Consequences Of obesity

Three categories may be used to describe the consequences of obesity: The state of one's physical, health, and social status
 Health
Individuals who are overweight or obese suffer from an elevated risk of the following:
Ailments of the coronary heart
An elevated blood pressure
Stroke (s)
Type 2 diabetes Some cancers
Experiencing fertility issues
Non-alcoholic fatty liver disease
In addition to the foregoing, obesity may shorten your life expectancy by up to 9 years and many chronic illnesses can be averted by keeping a healthy weight.
Carrying excess weight may also place extra strain on joints and limbs, making activities rather difficult, and occasionally, any movement can be uncomfortable.
In pregnancy, women with obesity have a greater risk of pregnancy than a healthy-weight woman.
Children and young people with obesity have the same health hazards as adults with obesity. Whilst symptoms

may not become obvious until later in life, in many situations, harm from childhood obesity has already been done, making it vitally crucial that children attain a healthy weight as early as possible. In truth, we are increasingly seeing youngsters with such extreme obesity that they are suffering from illnesses traditionally exclusively associated with adults e.g. Type 2 diabetes. But it's not all doom and gloom since there is aid available.

The fantastic news is that simply lowering body weight by only 5-10% drastically decreases health risks. Losing weight also implies levels of exercise may be increased - leading to additional weight reduction.

PSYCHOLOGICAL Studies have indicated that obesity may contribute to psychological disorders such as:Depression,Anxiety,Low quality of life,Low self-esteem,Body dissatisfaction

Studies have found that children with obesity rank their quality of life lower than those youngsters with cancer.

Weight increase has also been related to low focus levels, poor academic progress, and social marginalization in school.

SOCIAL Research shows us that persons with obesity might also have social challenges such as:

More likely to suffer from prejudice and discrimination in various settings (for example work, travel, education, healthcare, shopping, etc.) Fewer friends,Lower educational attainment

Lower employment

CHAPTER 1

WHAT CAUSED THE OBESITY EPIDERMIC?

Obesity is one of the most significant health issues that the globe encounters today.

It is linked to a number of disorders that are connected to one another and are collectively referred to as metabolic syndrome. For example, increased blood pressure, raised blood sugar, and an unsatisfactory blood lipid profile are all examples of these.

When compared to those whose weight is within the normal range, those who have metabolic syndrome are at a significantly increased risk of developing cardiovascular disease and type 2 diabetes.

It seems that a lot of individuals are under the impression that a lack of willpower is the root cause of weight gain and obesity.

That's not fully accurate. Despite the fact that eating habits and lifestyle choices are the primary contributors to weight gain, there are certain individuals who are at a disadvantage when it comes to exercising control over their food habits.

The reality of the matter is that excessive eating is caused by a number of biological variables, including hormones and heredity. Certain individuals just have a genetic predisposition to putting on weight.

Without a doubt, individuals are able to overcome the hereditary disadvantages they have by making adjustments to their lifestyle and conduct. Lifestyle changes need effort, focus, and patience.

Nevertheless, statements that conduct is entirely a result of willpower are much too simple.

They don't take into consideration all the other elements that ultimately decide what individuals do and when they do it.

Causes of Weight Gain and Obesity

1. Genetics

Obesity has a high hereditary component. Children whose parents are obese are far more likely to have obesity than children of lean parents.

That doesn't imply that obesity is fully predestined. What you consume may have a huge influence on which genes are expressed and which are not.

Non-industrialized civilizations quickly become obese when they start eating a standard Western diet. Their DNA didn't change, but the environment and the signals they transmitted to their genes changed.

Put simply, genetic components do increase your propensity to acquire weight. Studies on identical twins reveal this extremely clearly.

Summary Some individuals seem to be genetically sensitive to weight gain and obesity.

2. Engineered Junk Foods

Heavily processed meals are typically nothing more than refined components coupled with additives.

These items are meant to be inexpensive, stay long on the market, and taste so fantastically delicious that they are hard to refuse.

By making meals as appetizing as possible, food makers are striving to enhance sales. But they also encourage overeating.

Most processed foods nowadays don't resemble real foods at all. These are carefully developed items, meant to get consumers hooked.

Summary Stores are packed with packaged meals that are hard to resist. These products also increase overeating.

3. Food Addiction

Many sugar-sweetened, high-fat junk meals trigger the reward centers in your brain.

In fact, these meals are frequently linked to widely misused narcotics including alcohol, cocaine, nicotine, and cannabis.

Junk foods may induce addiction in vulnerable people. These individuals lose control over their eating habits, comparable to persons battling with alcohol addiction losing control over their drinking activity.

Addiction is a complicated condition that may be extremely tough to overcome. When you get addicted to anything, you lose your freedom of choice and the biochemistry in your brain begins calling the shots for you.

Summary Some individuals have extreme eating cravings or addiction. This notably applies to sugar-sweetened, high-fat junk meals which trigger the reward centers in the brain.

4. Aggressive Marketing

Junk food makers are incredibly active marketers.

Their techniques might turn dishonest at times and they occasionally attempt to pitch highly harmful items as healthy meals.

These firms also make deceptive promises. What's worse, they direct their advertisements exclusively to youngsters.

In today's environment, children are growing obese getting diabetic, and hooked to junk foods long before they're mature enough to make educated judgments about these things.

Summary Food makers spend a lot of money promoting bad food, often explicitly targeting youngsters, who don't have the knowledge and experience to recognize they are being deceived.

5. Insulin

Insulin is a highly essential hormone that controls energy storage, among other things.

One of its roles is to signal fat cells to store fat and hang on to the fat they currently contain.

The Western diet induces insulin resistance in many overweight and those with obesity. This boosts insulin levels all across the body, causing energy to be stored in fat cells instead of being accessible for utilization.

While insulin's function in obesity is debatable, some studies imply that elevated insulin levels have a causal impact on the development of obesity.

One of the greatest strategies to reduce your insulin is to cut down on simple or refined carbs while boosting fiber consumption.

This generally leads to a spontaneous decrease in calorie intake and uncomplicated weight loss – no calorie tracking or portion management is required.

Summary High insulin levels and insulin resistance are connected to the development of obesity. To decrease insulin levels, cut your consumption of refined carbohydrates and consume more fiber.

6. Certain Medications

Many pharmacological medicines might induce weight gain as a side effect.

For example, antidepressants have been related to mild weight increases over time.

Other examples are diabetic medicine and antipsychotics.

These medications don't reduce your willpower. They influence the operation of your body and brain, decreasing metabolic rate or raising hunger.

Summary Some drugs may cause weight gain by lowering the quantity of calories expended or boosting hunger.

7. Leptin Resistance

Leptin is another hormone that plays a significant function in obesity.

It is generated by fat cells and its blood levels rise with increased fat mass. For this reason, leptin levels are notably high in patients with obesity.

In healthy persons, increased leptin levels are connected to decreased appetite. When performing correctly, it should signal your brain how high your fat reserves are.

The trouble is that leptin isn't operating as it should in many individuals who are obese since for some reason it cannot penetrate the blood-brain barrier.

This syndrome is termed leptin resistance and is thought to play a key role in the pathophysiology of obesity.

Summary Leptin, an appetite-reducing hormone, doesn't function in many persons who have obesity.

8. Food Availability

Another element that greatly increases people's waistline is food availability, which has expanded tremendously in the previous several centuries.

Food, particularly junk food, is omnipresent today. Shops showcase appealing meals where they are most likely to attract your attention.

Another difficulty is that junk food is typically cheaper than nutritious, whole meals, particularly in America.

Some individuals, particularly in impoverished districts, don't even have the choice of buying actual goods, such as fresh fruit and vegetables.

Convenience shops in these locations exclusively offer drinks, candy, and processed packaged junk meals.

How can it be a question of choice if there is none?

Summary In certain locations, acquiring fresh, healthful meals may be difficult or costly, giving consumers little alternative except to purchase harmful junk foods.

9. Sugar

 Added sugar may be the single worst component of the contemporary diet.

That's because sugar alters the hormones and biochemistry of your body when taken in excess. This, in turn, adds to weight growth.

Added sugar is half glucose, half fructose. People receive glucose from a number of meals, including carbohydrates, but the bulk of fructose comes from added sugar.

Excess fructose consumption may promote insulin resistance and increased insulin levels. It also doesn't produce satiety in the same way glucose does.

For all these reasons, sugar leads to increased energy storage and, eventually, obesity.

Summary Scientists think that high sugar consumption may be one of the primary reasons for obesity.

10. Misinformation

People all across the globe are being deceived about health and nutrition.

There are various causes behind this, but the issue mostly hinges on where individuals acquire their information from.

Many websites, for example, transmit incomplete or even false information regarding health and diet.

Some news sources also oversimplify or misrepresent the outcomes of scientific research and the results are usually presented out of context.
Other information may simply be old or based on assumptions that have never been completely confirmed.

Food corporations also have a role. Some market things, such as weight reduction pills, that do not work.

Weight loss tactics based on erroneous information might hold back your progress. It's crucial to pick your sources properly.

Summary Misinformation may lead to weight gain in certain persons. It may also make weight reduction more challenging.

CHAPTER 2

THE HORMONAL MECHANISM OF OBESITY

Hormones are vital chemicals that function as chemical messengers in your body.

They promote practically every biological activity, including metabolism, appetite, and satiety. Because of their relationship with hunger, certain hormones also have a substantial effect on body weight.

9 hormones that may impact your weight, along with strategies for managing them at healthy levels.
1. Insulin

Insulin, the major storage hormone in your body, is generated by your pancreas. In healthy people, insulin stimulates the storage of glucose — a simple sugar you acquire from meals — in the muscle, liver, and fat cells for later use.

Your body secretes insulin in small quantities throughout the day and in bigger amounts after meals. This hormone then moves glucose from meals into your cells for either energy or storage, depending on your body's present demands.

Insulin resistance is a pretty frequent issue that causes your cells to cease reacting to insulin. This illness leads to elevated blood sugar because the insulin cannot transfer glucose into your cells.

Your pancreas subsequently creates even more insulin to improve glucose absorption.

Insulin resistance has been related to obesity, which in turn may have a role in other illnesses, such as type 2 diabetes and heart disease.

Insulin sensitivity may be thought of as the reverse of insulin resistance. It suggests your cells are responsive to insulin. Thus, it's a good idea to concentrate on lifestyle practices that help enhance insulin sensitivity, such as the following.

Tips to enhance insulin sensitivity

Exercise frequently. Research supports exercise, at both high and moderate intensities, as a technique for enhancing insulin sensitivity and lowering insulin resistance.

Improve your sleep patterns. Not getting enough sleep, or not receiving quality sleep, is connected to obesity and insulin resistance.

Get extra omega-3 fatty acids. Research shows that omega-3 supplementation may enhance insulin sensitivity in persons with metabolic disorders such as diabetes. If you aren't a fan of supplements, consider eating more fish, nuts, seeds, and plant oils.

Change your diet. The Mediterranean diet— which contains numerous vegetables, as well as healthful fats from nuts and extra-virgin olive oil — may help minimize insulin resistance. Decreasing your consumption of saturated and trans fats may also assist.

Maintain a reasonable weight. In those with overweight, good weight reduction and weight control may enhance insulin sensitivity.

Focus on low glycemic carbohydrates. Rather than attempt to remove carbohydrates from your diet, seek to make most of them low glycemic and high fiber. SUMMARY Insulin resistance is connected to chronic illnesses such as type 2 diabetes and heart disease. To enhance insulin sensitivity, concentrate on regular exercise, a nutritious diet, and better sleep patterns.

2. Leptin

Leptin is a fullness hormone that works by informing your hypothalamus — the area of your brain that controls hunger — that you're full.
However, those with obesity may suffer leptin resistance. This means the message to quit eating doesn't reach your brain, ultimately leading you to overeat.

As a result, your body may manufacture even more leptin until your levels become excessive.

The primary etiology of leptin resistance is unknown, however, it may be linked to inflammation, gene alterations, and/or increased leptin synthesis, which may occur with obesity.

Tips to boost leptin levels
Although no recognized therapy exists for leptin resistance, a few lifestyle adjustments may help reduce leptin levels:

Maintain a healthy weight. Because leptin resistance is related to obesity, it's crucial to maintain a healthy weight. Additionally, evidence shows that a reduction in body fat may help lower leptin levels.
Improve your sleep quality. Leptin levels may be connected to sleep quality in patients with obesity. Although this link may not exist in those without fat, there are various other reasons to gain better sleep.
Exercise frequently. Research relates regular, consistent exercise to a drop in leptin levels.

SUMMARY In patients with obesity, resistance to the hormone leptin, which helps you feel full, may contribute to overeating. Research shows that exercising frequently, resting properly, and keeping a healthy body weight can reduce leptin levels.

3. Ghrelin

Ghrelin is the reverse of leptin. It's the hunger hormone that sends a message to your brain signaling that your stomach is empty and requires food. Its major purpose is to promote hunger.

People with obesity have low ghrelin levels yet are more vulnerable to its effects. This sensitivity may lead to overeating.

Tips to control ghrelin levels

One reason weight reduction might be difficult is because reducing calories generally leads to higher ghrelin levels, keeping you hungry. Additionally, metabolism tends to slow down and leptin levels fall.

As such, here are some suggestions for reducing ghrelin to help decrease appetite:

Maintain a modest body weight. Obesity may raise your sensitivity to ghrelin, consequently boosting your hunger.

Try to obtain high-quality sleep.Because poor sleep may increase ghrelin, overeating, and weight gain.

Eat frequently.

 Because ghrelin levels are greatest before a meal, listen to your body and eat when you're hungry.

SUMMARY People with obesity may become more susceptible to the effects of the hunger hormone ghrelin. Research shows that keeping a healthy body weight and prioritizing sleep aid in controlling this hormone.

4. Cortisol

Cortisol is known as the stress hormone and is generated by your adrenal glands.

During times of stress, this hormone induces an increase in heart rate and energy levels. The production of cortisol — with the hormone adrenaline — is frequently dubbed the "fight or flight".

While it's vital for your to body release cortisol in hazardous conditions, persistent high amounts may lead to various health concerns, including heart disease, diabetes, poor energy levels, high blood pressure, sleep disruptions, and weight gain.

Certain lifestyle factors— including poor sleep patterns, prolonged stress, and large consumption of high glycemic meals — may lead to elevated cortisol levels.

Plus, not only can obesity elevate cortisol levels, but excessive levels may also induce weight growth, producing a negative feedback loop.

Tips for reducing cortisol levels

Here are some lifestyle adjustments that may help control cortisol levels:

Optimize sleep. Chronic sleep difficulties, including insomnia, sleep apnea, and irregular sleep patterns may lead to excessive cortisol levels. Focus on creating a consistent bedtime and sleep regimen.

Exercise frequently. Cortisol levels momentarily rise following high-intensity exercise, but regular exercise typically helps reduce levels by improving overall health and decreasing stress levels.

Practice mindfulness. study shows that frequently practicing mindfulness decreases cortisol levels, while additional study is required. Try incorporating meditation into your everyday regimen.

Maintain a modest body weight. Because obesity may raise cortisol levels and high cortisol levels may induce weight gain, keeping a healthy weight may help keep levels in balance.

Eat a balanced diet. Research has indicated that diets heavy in added sugars, processed carbohydrates, and saturated fat may contribute to greater cortisol levels. Additionally, adopting the Mediterranean diet may help reduce cortisol levels.

SUMMARY While cortisol is a vital hormone, persistently excessive levels may contribute to illnesses such as obesity, heart disease, and diabetes. Eating a balanced diet, exercising frequently, improving sleep, and practicing mindfulness may help reduce your levels.

5. Estrogen

Estrogen is a sex hormone involved in controlling the female reproductive system, as well as the immunological, skeletal, and circulatory systems.

Levels of this hormone alter throughout life phases such as pregnancy, lactation, and menopause, as well as during the menstrual cycle.

High levels of estrogen, which are typically present in persons with obesity, are connected with an increased risk of some malignancies and other chronic disorders.

Conversely, low levels — often found with age, perimenopause, and menopause — may impact body weight and body fat, thereby also raising your risk of chronic diseases.

Individuals with low estrogen levels commonly have central obesity, which is a buildup of weight around the trunk of the body. This may lead to various health concerns, such as excessive blood sugar, high blood pressure, and heart disease. You may minimize your risk of many of these health disorders by lifestyle changes — notably by keeping a healthy body weight.

Tips to maintain healthy estrogen levels

To maintain estrogen levels at a healthy balance, consider some of these techniques:

Try to regulate your weight. Weight reduction or maintenance may minimize the risk of heart disease owing to low estrogen levels in women aged 55–75. Research also supports optimal weight maintenance for minimizing the risk of chronic illnesses in general.

Exercise frequently. Low estrogen levels may leave you feeling less capable of working exercise. When estrogen is being produced in low amounts mostly during menopause, regular exercise is still helpful to promote weight control.

Follow a balanced diet. Diets strong in red meat, processed foods, sweets, and refined grains have been found to elevate estrogen levels, which may raise your risk of chronic illness. As such, you may desire to restrict your consumption of certain items.

SUMMARY Both high and low levels of the sex hormone estrogen may contribute to weight gain and eventually raise your risk of illness, so it's vital to maintain healthy lifestyle behaviors to keep these risks low.

6. Neuropeptide Y

Neuropeptide Y (NPY) is a hormone generated by cells in your brain and nervous system that increases hunger and reduces energy expenditure in response to fasting or stress. Because it may boost food intake, NPY is connected with obesity and weight gain.

It's triggered in fat tissue and may enhance fat accumulation and contribute to abdominal obesity and metabolic syndrome, a condition that may raise the risk of chronic illnesses. Research has demonstrated that NPY's pathways that contribute to obesity may also produce an inflammatory response, further exacerbating health issues.

Tips for keeping low NPY levels

Here are some suggestions for maintaining appropriate levels of NPY:

Exercise. Some studies show that regular exercise may help lower NPY levels, while data is inconsistent.

Eat a healthful diet. Although additional study is required, high-fat, high-sugar diets may boost NPY levels – thus you may want to try limiting your consumption of meals heavy in sugar and fat.

SUMMARY NPY is an appetite-stimulating hormone that may contribute to obesity. To maintain healthy levels, it may be useful to exercise often and eat appropriately.

7. Glucagon-like peptide-1

Glucagon-like peptide-1 (GLP-1) is a hormone generated in your gut when foods enter your intestines. It serves a vital role in maintaining blood sugar levels constant and helping you feel full.

Research shows that patients with obesity may have difficulties with GLP-1 signaling.

As such, GLP-1 is added to drugs — notably for those with diabetes — to lower body weight and waist circumference.

Tips for keeping GLP-1 levels under control

Here are some strategies to help maintain appropriate levels of GLP-1:

Eat lots of protein. High protein diets such as whey protein and yogurt have been demonstrated to boost GLP-1 levels.

Consider taking probiotics. Preliminary study shows that probiotics may enhance GLP-1 levels, while further human research is required. Additionally, it's advisable to consult with a healthcare expert before taking any new supplements.

SUMMARY

GLP-1 is a fullness hormone, although those with obesity may not be as susceptible to its effects. To maintain appropriate

GLP-1 levels, strive to eat a well-rounded diet with enough of protein.

8. Cholecystokinin

Like GLP-1, cholecystokinin (CCK) is a fullness hormone released by cells in your stomach after a meal. It's necessary for energy generation, protein synthesis, digestion, and other biological activities.

Those who are obese may have a reduced sensitivity to CCK's effects, which may lead to overeating. In turn,creating a negative feedback loop.

Tips for increasing CCK levels

Eat lots of protein. This may help increase CCK levels, and therefore fullness.

Exercise. While research is limited, some evidence supports regular exercise for boosting CCK levels.

SUMMARY CCK is a fullness hormone that persons with obesity may develop sensitivity to. This may lead to overeating. Consider frequent exercise and a diet with enough of protein to maintain appropriate CCK levels.

9. Peptide YY

Peptide YY (PYY) is another gastrointestinal hormone that lowers hunger.

PYY levels may be reduced in patients with obesity, and this may contribute to a larger hunger and overeating. Sufficient levels are considered to have a vital impact in limiting food consumption and minimizing the risk of obesity.

Tips for boosting PYY levels

Here are several strategies to maintain PYY at a healthy level in your body:

Follow a well-rounded diet. Eating lots of protein may encourage appropriate PYY levels and satiety. Additionally, the paleo diet — which contains adequate protein, fruits, and vegetables — may enhance PYY levels, although additional study is required.

Exercise. While data on exercise and PYY levels are conflicting, being active is usually helpful for health.

SUMMARY People with obesity may have decreased levels of the satiety hormone PYY. Eating a high-protein diet and being active may help boost levels.

CHAPTER 3

THE CALORIE CONUNDRUM

A calorie is a unit of energy corresponding to about 4.1868 joules of energy and is informally defined as the amount of heat required to raise the temperature of a quantity of water by one degree.

All nutritive foods contain calories and our ability to convert that energy into another usable form of energy within the body is the reason (quite simply) that we are alive and the reason our bodies can perform all physical and physiological tasks, including breathing, digesting food, thinking and moving.

The quantity of energy meals give is generally expressed in thousands of calories (kilocalories or kcal). However, people generally use the phrase "calories" instead, because "kilocalories" is an unpleasant word to use!

There are several reasons why you may choose to take a long hard look at calorie tracking as a tactic for reaching your objectives or improving your health situations.

Why We're Terrible at Losing Weight

Calorie counting is challenging, but it doesn't have to be. Losing weight sounds so straightforward: eat fewer calories than you burn. Easy, right? Yet, why do so many of us struggle to drop those additional pounds? Countless individuals limit calories and even monitor their meals using food tracking apps, only to feel disheartened when they don't observe any improvements on the scale. Frustrated with halted weight reduction, individuals typically blame things beyond their control: a slow metabolism or adverse genetic predispositions. However, the harsh fact is that it's probably not their genes or their metabolisms; most individuals struggle with precisely managing calories. These tiny flaws are frequent enough to ruin any amount of hard effort. Let's take a look at why this occurs and what we can do.

1. Hidden Calories in Unseen Ingredients

One of the key culprits in our caloric misunderstanding is a lack of information about what's in our food and how it's cooked, particularly when eating out. Restaurants commonly employ fattier cuts of meat and significant quantities of sugar, butter, and/or oil to enhance tastes. This culinary innovation could make our taste sense, but it also adds a huge calorie weight to our meals. These harmless approaches, such as adding bacon to meals, enhancing veggies with butter, and infusing sauces with oil and sugar, each contribute up to an additional 200 calories per serving. Yet, it's the aggregate impact of these hidden calorie increases in every component of our meal that offers the main issue in determining the total caloric intake.

2. Portion Distortion

Distorted portion sizes constitute a huge challenge to effectively measuring our calorie consumption, whether it is at restaurants or with premade meals. Consider a basic pasta meal featured on a menu as a single serving. Yet, what appears on your plate is an amount designed for three or four people – a regular occurrence in both restaurant portions and many frozen premade meals.

The disparity goes beyond food portions; it also extends to the substances utilized in our meals. Consider the standard grilled cheese sandwich — a package label would say 100 calories for a single serving of cheese, normally equivalent to a solitary slice. There's a widespread instinctive assumption that a meal made for one would only include one portion of every component. However, reality tends to be considerably different, as restaurants and many customers choose three slices, doubling the predicted cheese calories without a second thought.

3. Neglecting the Power of Food Labels

Information on food labels sometimes goes missing. Understanding the calorie composition of your diet is crucial for weight reduction. Not only do most individuals ignore these facts, but they also lack understanding about the fat or carbohydrate levels in different meals. Consequently, even if told to 'avoid carbs' or 'limit saturated fat,' many would struggle, uninformed of how to identify and control these items in their diet. For instance, the harmless 16-ounce bag of chips, seen as a single meal, really translates to three servings according to the label. Even more troubling is the fact that some folks don't even realize that chips are deep-fried and particularly heavy in fat! Neglecting these crucial facts might unwittingly lead to ingesting extra calories, derailing your weight reduction attempts while offering a false feeling of nutritional stability.

Improving Your Accuracy

Improving the precision of calorie monitoring is crucial for weight reduction. A key initial step is reviewing food labels for all substances or meals ingested. Paying attention to the calories, macronutrients, and serving sizes mentioned on labels is vital. You'll be astonished to discover how little actual serving sizes may be. Take peanut butter, for instance – although 2 tablespoons may sound substantial, it's nearly the size of a golf ball. Yet, without measuring, it's simple to mistakenly exceed the desired portion, unwittingly ingesting more calories than expected. Peanut butter, in particular, is infamous for being calorie-dense; just a tiny margin of error in calculating quantities may result to a considerable caloric excess.

Measuring out correct servings is the next stage in mastering calorie counting. Investing in a dependable kitchen scale or measuring cups is crucial to precisely measure servings. Precise measurements offer a clear knowledge of your calorie consumption. It's a minor tweak that delivers enormous insights into the real calorie composition of your meals. While this may seem like overkill, it is vital to do this until you get accustomed to what a portion size should look like. By constantly measuring amounts initially, you get a genuine grasp of serving sizes, enabling you to better estimate and regulate your intake even without the use of scales or measuring cups in the long term.

For most of us, as long as calories are actually below calories burnt, reducing those excess pounds is within grasp. But the true problem comes in ensuring that the calories we imagine we're ingesting coincide with reality.

While reading labels and painstakingly measuring every element of your meal can sound onerous and cumbersome, these activities are the keystones to ensuring that our calorie intake coincides with our weight reduction objectives. It's this attention to detail that changes our path from a simple numbers game into a blueprint to success.

By being conscious of portion sizes and measuring our food consumption precisely, we can make educated judgments about our nutrition and make modifications as required. Additionally, knowing the nutritional worth of the foods we eat may help us make better choices and maximize our weight reduction journey.

CHAPTER 4

STRUCTURING A DIET FOR SUSTAINABLE WEIGHT LOSS

Meal planning may be a beneficial tool if you're attempting to lose weight.

When done appropriately, it may help you achieve the calorie deficit essential for weight reduction while offering your body the nutritional meals it needs to operate and stay healthy.

Planning your meals may help simplify the meal prep process and save you time.

This article discusses the most crucial components of meal planning for weight reduction, including a few simple recipes and additional ideas to help you attain your objectives.

How to meal plan for weight loss

When it comes to weight reduction meal plans, the enormity of possibilities might be intimidating. Here are a few things to bear in mind while you look for the most suited plan.

Creating a calorie deficit in a nutrient-dense method

All weight reduction strategies have one thing in common – they get you to consume less calories than you burn.

However, whilst a calorie deficit can help you lose weight regardless of how it's formed, what you eat is just as essential as how much you consume. That's because the dietary choices you make are crucial in helping you satisfy your nutritional demands.

A decent weight reduction meal plan should meet several common criteria:

Includes lots of protein and fiber. Protein- and fiber-rich meals can keep you fuller for longer, lowering cravings and helping you feel pleased with fewer servings.

Limits processed foods and added sugar. Rich in calories but poor in nutrients, these meals fail to activate satiety regions in your brain and make it difficult to shed weight or satisfy your nutritional demands.

Includes a range of fruits and veggies. Both are rich in water and fiber, leading to feelings of fullness. These nutrient-rich meals also make it easy to achieve your daily nutritional needs.

Building nutrient-dense meals

To include these recommendations in your weight reduction meal plan, start by filling one-third to one-half of your plate with non-starchy veggies. These are low in calories and give water, fiber, and many of the vitamins and minerals you need.

Then, fill one-quarter to one-third of your plate with protein-rich meals, such as meat, fish, tofu, seitan, or legumes, and the remaining with nutritious grains, fruit, or starchy vegetables. These offer protein, vitamins, minerals, and additional fiber. You may increase the taste of your dish with a splash of healthy fats from foods like avocados, olives, nuts, and seeds. Some individuals may benefit from eating a snack to tide their hunger over between meals. Protein- and fiber-rich snacks appear the most helpful for weight reduction.

Good examples are apple slices with peanut butter, veggies and hummus, roasted chickpeas, or Greek yogurt with fruit and almonds.

SUMMARY

An effective weight reduction meal plan should establish a calorie deficit while addressing your dietary demands.

Helpful suggestions to make meal planning work for you

An essential part of a good weight reduction meal plan is its capacity to help you keep the lost weight off.

Here are some strategies to assist boost your food plan's long-term sustainability.

Pick a meal-planning technique that matches your schedule

There are different methods to meal plan, so be sure to select the approach that best matches your lifestyle.

You may opt to batch cook all of your meals over the weekend, so you can conveniently take individual pieces during the week. Alternatively, you may want to cook every day, in which case, selecting to prep all of your items ahead of time would work best for you.

If you don't enjoy following recipes or want a little more freedom, you may opt for a technique that demands you to stock your refrigerator and pantry with specified quantities of ingredients each week while allowing you to improvise when putting them together for meals.

Batch shopping for groceries is another wonderful method that helps save time while keeping your refrigerator and pantry packed with nutrient-dense items.

Consider testing an app

Apps may be a great tool in your meal-planning arsenal. Some applications include meal plan templates that you may edit depending on your dietary choices or sensitivities. They may also be a helpful tool to keep track of your favorite recipes and preserve all of your data in one spot.

What's more, several apps give tailored shopping lists based on your preferred recipes or what's left over in your fridge, helping you save time and decrease food waste.

Pick enough recipes

Picking a suitable amount of recipes guarantees that you have enough diversity without needing to spend all of your leisure time in the kitchen.

When determining how many meals to cook, look at your schedule to assess the amount of times you're likely to dine out — whether for a date, client dinner, or brunch with friends.

Divide the remaining number of breakfasts, lunches, and dinners by the number of meals that you can reasonably cook or prepare for that week. This helps you decide the amounts of each meal you'll need to prep.

Then, just search through your cookbooks or internet food blogs to find your recipes.

Consider snacks

Allowing yourself to feel extremely hungry between meals may lead you to overeat at your next meal, making it more difficult to attain your weight reduction objectives.

Snacks may help suppress hunger, enhance feelings of fullness, and reduce the total amount of calories you consume each day.

Protein- and fiber-rich combos, such as almonds, roasted chickpeas, or vegetables and hummus, look most adapted to assist weight reduction.

However, bear in mind that some individuals tend to gain weight when adding snacks to their meals. So make sure you check your outcomes while employing this method.

Ensure variety

Eating a variety of meals is crucial in giving your body the nutrients it needs.

That's why it's better to avoid meal plans that propose batch preparing 1–2 meals for the full week. This lack of diversity might make it difficult to achieve your daily dietary requirements and lead to boredom over time, lowering your meal plan's sustainability.

Instead, ensure that your meal contains a variety of items each day.

Speed up your meal prep time

Meal planning doesn't have to involve lengthy hours in the kitchen. Here are a few strategies to speed up your dinner prep time.

Stick to a regimen. Picking certain times to plan the week's meals, shopping shop, and prepare may simplify your decision-making process and make your meal-planning process more effective.

Grocery shop using a list. Detailed food lists may minimize your shopping time. Try structuring your list by grocery sections to minimize going back to a previously visited sector.

Pick suitable recipes. When batch cooking, pick recipes that employ various equipment. For instance, one dish may need the oven, no more than two burners on the cooktop, and no heating at all.

Schedule your cook times. Organize your workflow by beginning with the dish needing the longest cooking time, then concentrate on the others. Electric pressure cookers or slow cookers may further minimize cooking times.

Inexperienced chefs or those just looking to decrease the time spent in the kitchen may opt to select meals that may be made in 15–20 minutes from start to finish.

Store and reheat your food securely

Storing and reheating your meals correctly may help retain their taste and limit your risk of food illness.

Here are some food safety rules to bear in mind.

Cook food thoroughly. Most meats should achieve an interior temperature of at least 165°F (75°C) during cooking since this destroys most pathogens.

Thaw food in the refrigerator. Thawing frozen foods or meals on your countertop might encourage germs to proliferate. If you're short on time, immerse meals in cold water, changing the water every 30 minutes.

Reheat food securely. Make careful to reheat your food to at least 165°F (75°C) before eating. Frozen meals should be consumed within 24 hours after defrosting.

Dispose of old food. Refrigerated meals should be eaten within 3–4 days after being cooked, and frozen meals should be consumed within 3–6 months.

SUMMARY

Picking a meal-planning strategy that works for you, coupled with an acceptable quantity and diversity of meals and snacks that can be prepared or reheated quickly and safely, boosts your probability of lasting weight reduction.

Easy recipe ideas

Weight loss recipes don't have to be extremely difficult. Here are a few easy-to-prepare recipes that demand a minimum amount of components.

Soups. Soups may be batch-cooked and frozen in individual quantities. Be sure to incorporate a lot of veggies, as well as meat, fish, beans, peas, or lentils. Add brown rice, quinoa, or potatoes if preferred.

Homemade pizza.

Salads. Salads are fast and adaptable. Start with leafy greens, a few colorful veggies, and a source of protein.

Pasta. Start with a whole-grain pasta of your choosing and a source of protein, such as chicken, fish, or tofu. Then combine a tomato-based spaghetti sauce or pesto and some veggies like broccoli or spinach.

Slow cooker or electric pressure cooker recipes. These are wonderful for preparing chili, enchiladas, spaghetti sauce, and stew. Simply insert your ingredients into your gadget, start it, and let it do all the work for you.

Grain bowls. Batch prepare grains like quinoa or brown rice then top with your choice of protein, such as chicken or hard-boiled eggs, non-starchy vegetables, and a healthy dressing of your taste.

SUMMARY

The recipe ideas above are easy and need very little time to create. They may also be cooked in many ways, making them highly adaptable.

Just bear in mind that fully omitting a food category may require you to take supplements to achieve your daily nutritional requirements.

SUMMARY

Weight-reduction meals should be nutrient-dense and high in protein and fiber. This meal plan may be altered for several dietary limitations but may need you to take supplements if fully eliminating a food group.

The bottom line
A solid weight reduction meal plan provides a calorie deficit while supplying all the nutrients you need.

Done well, it can be really easy and save you a lot of time. Picking a strategy that works for you might also lower your risk of regaining weight. All-in-all, meal planning is an exceptionally effective weight reduction strategy.

CHAPTER 3
THE CALORIE CONUNDRUM
A calorie is a unit of energy corresponding to about 4.1868 joules of energy and is informally defined as the amount of heat required to raise the temperature of a quantity of water by one degree.
All nutritive foods contain calories and our ability to convert that energy into another usable form of energy within the

body is the reason (quite simply) that we are alive and the reason our bodies can perform all physical and physiological tasks, including breathing, digesting food, thinking, and moving.

The quantity of energy meals give is generally expressed in thousands of calories (kilocalories or kcal). However, people generally use the phrase "calories" instead, because "kilocalories" is an unpleasant word to use!
There are several reasons why you may choose to take a long hard look at calorie tracking as a tactic for reaching your objectives or improving your health situations.

Why We're Terrible at Losing Weight

Calorie counting is challenging, but it doesn't have to be. Losing weight sounds so straightforward: eat fewer calories than you burn. Easy, right? Yet, why do so many of us struggle to drop those additional pounds? Countless individuals limit calories and even monitor their meals using food tracking apps, only to feel disheartened when they don't observe any improvements on the scale. Frustrated with halted weight reduction, individuals typically blame things beyond their control: a slow metabolism or adverse genetic predispositions. However, the harsh fact is that it's probably not their genes or their metabolisms; most individuals struggle with precisely managing calories. These tiny flaws are frequent enough to ruin any amount of hard effort. Let's take a look at why this occurs and what we can do.

1. Hidden Calories in Unseen Ingredients

One of the key culprits in our caloric misunderstanding is a lack of information about what's in our food and how it's cooked, particularly when eating out. Restaurants commonly employ fattier cuts of meat and significant quantities of sugar, butter, and/or oil to enhance tastes. This culinary innovation could make our taste sense, but it also adds a huge calorie weight to our meals. These harmless approaches, such as adding bacon to meals, enhancing veggies with butter, and infusing sauces with oil and sugar, each contribute up to an additional 200 calories per serving. Yet, it's the aggregate impact of these hidden calorie increases in every component of our meal that offers the main issue in determining the total caloric intake.

2. Portion Distortion

Distorted portion sizes constitute a huge challenge to effectively measuring our calorie consumption, whether it is at restaurants or with premade meals. Consider a basic pasta meal featured on a menu as a single serving. Yet, what appears on your plate is an amount designed for three or four people – a regular occurrence in both restaurant portions and many frozen premade meals.

The disparity goes beyond food portions; it also extends to the substances utilized in our meals. Consider the standard grilled cheese sandwich — a package label would say 100 calories for a single serving of cheese, normally equivalent to a solitary slice. There's a widespread instinctive assumption that a meal made for one would only include one portion of every component. However, reality tends to be considerably different, as restaurants and many customers choose three slices, doubling the predicted cheese calories without a second thought.

3. Neglecting the Power of Food Labels

Information on food labels sometimes goes missing. Understanding the calorie composition of your diet is crucial for weight reduction. Not only do most individuals ignore these facts, but they also lack understanding about the fat or carbohydrate levels in different meals. Consequently, even if told to 'avoid carbs' or 'limit saturated fat,' many would struggle, uninformed of how to identify and control these items in their diet. For instance, the harmless 16-ounce bag of chips, seen as a single meal, really translates to three servings according to the label. Even more troubling is the fact that some folks don't even realize that chips are deep-fried and particularly heavy in fat! Neglecting these crucial facts might unwittingly lead to ingesting extra calories, derailing your weight reduction attempts while offering a false feeling of nutritional stability.

Improving Your Accuracy

Improving the precision of calorie monitoring is crucial for weight reduction. A key initial step is reviewing food labels for all substances or meals ingested. Paying attention to the calories, macronutrients, and serving sizes mentioned on labels is vital. You'll be astonished to discover how little actual serving sizes may be. Take peanut butter, for instance – although 2 tablespoons may sound substantial, it's nearly the size of a golf ball. Yet, without measuring, it's simple to mistakenly exceed the desired portion, unwittingly ingesting more calories than expected. Peanut butter, in particular, is infamous for being calorie-dense; just a tiny margin of error in calculating quantities may result in considerable caloric excess.

Measuring out correct servings is the next stage in mastering calorie counting. Investing in a dependable kitchen scale or measuring cups is crucial to precisely measure servings. Precise measurements offer a clear knowledge of your calorie consumption. It's a minor tweak that delivers enormous insights into the real calorie composition of your meals. While this may seem like overkill, it is vital to do this until you get accustomed to what a portion size should look like. By constantly measuring amounts initially, you get a genuine grasp of serving sizes, enabling you to better estimate and regulate your intake even without the use of scales or measuring cups in the long term.

For most of us, as long as calories are actually below calories burnt, reducing those excess pounds is within grasp. But the true problem comes in ensuring that the calories we imagine we're ingesting coincide with reality.

While reading labels and painstakingly measuring every element of your meal can sound onerous and cumbersome, these activities are the keystones to ensuring that our calorie intake coincides with our weight reduction objectives. It's this attention to detail that changes our path from a simple numbers game into a blueprint to success.

By being conscious of portion sizes and measuring our food consumption precisely, we can make educated judgments about our nutrition and make modifications as required. Additionally, knowing the nutritional worth of the foods we eat may help us make better choices and maximize our weight reduction journey.

CHAPTER 4
STRUCTURING A DIET FOR SUSTAINABLE WEIGHT LOSS

Meal planning may be a beneficial tool if you're attempting to lose weight.

When done appropriately, it may help you achieve the calorie deficit essential for weight reduction while offering your body the nutritional meals it needs to operate and stay healthy.

Planning your meals may help simplify the meal prep process and save you time.

This article discusses the most crucial components of meal planning for weight reduction, including a few simple recipes and additional ideas to help you attain your objectives.

How to meal plan for weight loss

When it comes to weight reduction meal plans, the enormity of possibilities might be intimidating. Here are a few things to bear in mind while you look for the most suited plan.

Creating a calorie deficit in a nutrient-dense method

All weight reduction strategies have one thing in common – they get you to consume less calories than you burn.

However, whilst a calorie deficit can help you lose weight regardless of how it's formed, what you eat is just as essential as how much you consume. That's because the dietary choices you make are crucial in helping you satisfy your nutritional demands.

A decent weight reduction meal plan should meet several common criteria:

Includes lots of protein and fiber. Protein- and fiber-rich meals can keep you fuller for longer, lowering cravings and helping you feel pleased with fewer servings.

Limits processed foods and added sugar. Rich in calories but poor in nutrients, these meals fail to activate satiety regions in your brain and make it difficult to shed weight or satisfy your nutritional demands.

Includes a range of fruits and veggies. Both are rich in water and fiber, leading to feelings of fullness. These nutrient-rich meals also make it easy to achieve your daily nutritional needs.

Building nutrient-dense meals

To include these recommendations in your weight reduction meal plan, start by filling one-third to one-half of your plate with non-starchy veggies. These are low in calories and give water, fiber, and many of the vitamins and minerals you need. Then, fill one-quarter to one-third of your plate with protein-rich meals, such as meat, fish, tofu, seitan, or legumes, and the remaining with nutritious grains, fruit, or starchy vegetables. These offer protein, vitamins, minerals, and additional fiber. You may increase the taste of your dish with a splash of healthy fats from foods like avocados, olives, nuts, and seeds. Some individuals may benefit from eating a snack to tide their hunger over between meals. Protein- and fiber-rich snacks appear the most helpful for weight reduction.

Good examples are apple slices with peanut butter, veggies and hummus, roasted chickpeas, or Greek yogurt with fruit and almonds.

SUMMARY

An effective weight reduction meal plan should establish a calorie deficit while addressing your dietary demands. Helpful suggestions to make meal planning work for you

An essential part of a good weight reduction meal plan is its capacity to help you keep the lost weight off.

Here are some strategies to assist boost your food plan's long-term sustainability.

Pick a meal-planning technique that matches your schedule There are different methods to meal plan, so be sure to select the approach that best matches your lifestyle.

You may opt to batch cook all of your meals over the weekend, so you can conveniently take individual pieces during the week. Alternatively, you may want to cook everyday, in which case, selecting to prep all of your items ahead of time would work best for you.

If you don't enjoy following recipes or want a little more freedom, you may opt for a technique that demands you to stock your refrigerator and pantry with specified quantities of ingredients each week while allowing you to improvise when putting them together for meals.

Batch shopping for groceries is another wonderful method that helps save time while keeping your refrigerator and pantry packed with nutrient-dense items.

Consider testing an app Apps may be a great tool in your meal-planning arsenal. Some applications include meal plan templates that you may edit depending on your dietary choices or sensitivities. They may also be a helpful tool to keep track of your favorite recipes and preserve all of your data in one spot.

What's more, several apps give tailored shopping lists based on your preferred recipes or what's left over in your fridge, helping you save time and decrease food waste.

Pick enough recipes

Picking a suitable amount of recipes guarantees that you have enough diversity without needing to spend all of your leisure time in the kitchen.

When determining how many meals to cook, look at your schedule to assess the amount of times you're likely to dine out — whether for a date, client dinner, or brunch with friends.

Divide the remaining number of breakfasts, lunches, and dinners by the number of meals that you can reasonably cook or prepare for that week. This helps you decide the amounts of each meal you'll need to prep.

Then, just search through your cookbooks or internet food blogs to find your recipes.

Consider snacks

Allowing yourself to feel extremely hungry between meals may lead you to overeat at your next meal, making it more difficult to attain your weight reduction objectives.

Snacks may help suppress hunger, enhance feelings of fullness, and reduce the total amount of calories you consume each day.

Protein- and fiber-rich combos, such as almonds, roasted chickpeas, or vegetables and hummus, look most adapted to assist weight reduction.

However, bear in mind that some individuals tend to gain weight when adding snacks to their meals. So make sure you check your outcomes while employing this method.

Ensure variety
Eating a variety of meals is crucial in giving your body the nutrients it needs.

That's why it's better to avoid meal plans that propose batch preparing 1–2 meals for the full week. This lack of diversity might make it difficult to achieve your daily dietary requirements and lead to boredom over time, lowering your meal plan's sustainability.

Instead, ensure that your meal contains a variety of items each day.

Speed up your meal prep time
Meal planning doesn't have to involve lengthy hours in the kitchen. Here are a few strategies to speed up your dinner prep time.

Stick to a regimen. Picking certain times to plan the week's meals, shop shop, and prepare may simplify your decision-making process and make your meal-planning process more effective.
Grocery shop using a list. Detailed food lists may minimize your shopping time. Try structuring your list by grocery sections to minimize going back to a previously visited sector.

Pick suitable recipes. When batch cooking, pick recipes that employ various equipment. For instance, one dish may need the oven, no more than two burners on the cooktop, and no heating at all.

Schedule your cook times. Organize your workflow by beginning with the dish needing the longest cooking time, then concentrate on the others. Electric pressure cookers or slow cookers may further minimize cooking times.

Inexperienced chefs or those just looking to decrease the time spent in the kitchen may opt to select meals that may be made in 15–20 minutes from start to finish.

Store and reheat your food securely

Storing and reheating your meals correctly may help retain their taste and limit your risk of food illness.

Here are some government-approved food safety rules to bear in mind (16, 17):

Cook food thoroughly. Most meats should achieve an interior temperature of at least 165°F (75°C) during cooking since this destroys most pathogens.

Thaw food in the refrigerator. Thawing frozen foods or meals on your countertop might encourage germs to proliferate. If you're short on time, immerse meals in cold water, changing the water every 30 minutes.

Reheat food securely. Make careful to reheat your food to at least 165°F (75°C) before eating. Frozen meals should be consumed within 24 hours after defrosting.

Dispose of old food. Refrigerated meals should be eaten within 3–4 days after being cooked, and frozen meals should be consumed within 3–6 months.

SUMMARY

Picking a meal-planning strategy that works for you, coupled with an acceptable quantity and diversity of meals and snacks that can be prepared or reheated quickly and safely, boosts your probability of lasting weight reduction.

9 798322 969143